MASSAGE MARKETING - BOOST PROFITS

SABRINA TONNESON

CONTENTS

INTRODUCTION

Most massage therapists embark on their careers with one fundamental motivation, a deep desire to help and heal others with massage therapy.

They plough their heart, soul, muscle and sinew into their careers and customers, yet they don't always harvest an income reflecting all they've invested in their business. Many of them are burdened with being overworked and underpaid.

Even though you are drawn to a deeper calling, the vocation of healing hands, you can't very well deposit feelings of Zen and inner peace at the bank.

You may be wondering; how can you hang a price tag on big heartedness? Healing compassion can't be quantified in dollars and cents, can it?

Even with all my considerable experience, I can't do that. What I can do, though, is help you shake up your business, making it more productive, efficient and lucrative.

Indeed, the purpose of this book is to help you, as a massage therapist, perceive what you do as a legitimate business. With the application of the principles detailed in this book, you can achieve a more favorable work-to-income balance, making your massage therapy as rewarding for you as it is for your clients.

This book asks and answers some important questions. How do you select prices for your massage practice? Why is undercharging a mistake? How can a business leverage more revenue with proper pricing? Why is your menu one of the most important pieces of your marketing? How does implementing a menu grow your business?

It's something that's easy to overlook, but a strategic menu is the most effective marketing maneuver of any massage practice.

This book will show you how to construct a menu that is a painless path to boosting profits without additional investments of time and money. Inside this book, you'll find step-by-step instructions for a profit-boosting business menu.

With a menu in hand, you can determine the best pricing. This is a critical step because pricing your services appropriately allows you to earn more while working less.

In here, you'll find worksheets and formulas to assist in the design and creation of your massage therapy services.

This book will teach you how to accelerate business growth by offering a variety of services.

Failing to charge properly for your work is like walking away from money. A menu detailing your services is a cost-free way to market your business, lure new customers and lock in all important repeat clients.

Every massage practice can benefit from this marketing tool, regardless of the size of your business.

My name is Sabrina Tonneson and I have over two decades of massage therapy experience. My practice had its humble beginnings in my home. Working from home, though, was more complicated than I had pictured in my head! Soon enough, I transplanted my fledgling operation to a rented room. Success quickly beckoned, so I leased my own space and expanded the business by hiring staff.

Over the years of owning and managing a massage therapy practice, I've discovered through trial and error, how to pilot a successful enterprise. Admittedly, one of my greatest challenges was mental fatigue.

At one point, my drive and enthusiasm cooled to crippling ennui. In addition to demotivation, burnout became a steady, unwelcome companion. I needed some kick-in-the-butt stimulation, and that came in the way of new services, new techniques and new marketing approaches.

My passion is creating business success. I've been mentoring individual businesses and companies for over 10 years.

Take it from me, running your own business means you need to be like an octopus, with many tentacles efficiently conducting different functions. I can help you cut an easy path to success.

It's my mission to guide massage therapists to achieve balance and distil appreciation and healthy compensation from hard work.

This book is dedicated to all of you with selfless hearts, nurturing souls, and sainted hands. If you follow the simple formulas and effective marketing tools contained in this book, you'll be assured of greater financial rewards for your talents.

WHY CREATE A BUSINESS MENU?

Proper pricing and a strategic menu are oxygen to any service-oriented business.

A fatal flaw of many massage therapists is the one service (massage therapy) one flat rate' mindset. That is a proven recipe for short-changing yourself. Even as a solo entrepreneur, a solid menu will transform your business. You need to design an effective menu to function as a blueprint for your pricing structure.

Before we delve into pricing, let's first focus on the importance of a menu. Massage therapy clients come from all walks of life. An understanding of your client demographics is the foundation of a services menu that checks every box in your client pool.

I'm going to describe some of the typical massage therapy clients coming across your table. Try to think of them like exotic birds.

There's the "I need to get a massage NOW!" customer. For this species of client, cost is of little consequence. The customer who needs a massage like an asthmatic needs an inhaler is willing to pay extra if you extend your hours to fit them in. Availability, not price, is their priority.

Then there's the "I'll shop around for a better deal" customer. This species is identified by their behavioral patterns, popping up when you dangle specials or low prices out there. They're most abundant during the sale season and are willing to schedule early in the morning or late in the evening. This customer's priority is snagging a bargain.

Another type of customer is the regular. This client is already sold on the benefits of a weekly or monthly massage. This particular species is searching for a life- mate, a massage therapist with the desired skill set. In the massage client world, this customer is, perhaps, the most sought-after species of them all. Stay with me on the exotic birds' analogy here!

And, of course, you have the high roller client. This peacock-like customer, for whom money is no object, is accustomed to being pampered. This species is known for strutting about and doing things like scheduling your deluxe packages. They want the best you can offer, while they drift off in a gentle current of serenity conjured by your spellbinding hands. That's the spare- no expense client.

Those are just a few of the customers that massage therapists encounter. Most businesses cater to a varied clientele so their menus and prices reflect this diversity.

Hotels are an excellent example of this pricing strategy. They apply higher nightly rates during peak periods and modest rates when demand slows. This follows the natural cycles of tourism seasons.

As a budget-conscious traveler, you probably vacation during the low season. If you are a high-end consumer, though, you'd likely book the most luxurious hotel suite, peak season or not. Similarly, restaurants have early bird dinner specials or happy hour specials. Such deals target the budget consumer willing to patronize their business during periods of slowed diner traffic.

Smart marketers create a variety of items on their menu. Your massage or service can benefit from the same marketing strategy.

If you can get past the thinking that you offer one basic item at a flat rate, you'll harness a huge marketing advantage and grow your practice double-time! You can attract a variety of customers with a menu designed to cater to their needs, wants and budgets.

Keep in mind, you can continue to massage that long-term goal of a specialization that most fits your preferences. A varied menu can help grow your practice at a faster pace, getting you closer to your ultimate business objectives. As appointments become filled and your customer base expands, you can adjust your marketing approach. Dropping services from your menu is always an option. You are the creator of your business, the captain of your destiny.

PRICING MISTAKES

So, I've already identified the 'one service, one price' pitfall common to many massage therapists. These businesses are too hasty in fixing their prices. Insufficient thought and strategy have gone into the process. Sometimes a business practitioner assumes if they charge the going rate in their area, then that's good enough.

Pricing, though, should be practiced as a function of marketing. Often, businesses start out hot and heavy, realizing shortly afterwards that their prices are too low. There you are with marketing and business materials already printed and the figures are depressingly off base. That can put you in a very tight spot. Penciling in new prices early in the life of a business can douse customers' interest. Instead of alienating customers, or flushing dollars down the tubes on printed materials, put in some time on research. Read this book and do the worksheets.

Have you heard the story of the two tree cutters, Tom and Larry? Every day Tom and Larry went to the woods to cut dead branches and fell dead trees. Larry spent several hours every day pruning trees. His neighbor, Tom, spent less time on the same task. One day Larry asked Tom how he manages to finish his tasks so quickly. Tom responded, "I prepare the saw in advance." Larry jumped in, exclaiming, "I don't have time to waste on preparing my saw!" Tom smiled and gently said, "Preparing the saw sharpens the blade. A sharp blade allows me to cut easily and effectively. A sharp blade allows me to finish quickly."

So, do you sharpen your blades before you start sawing your customers? Wait, I've taken the analogy a bit too far! Ask yourself: do you sharpen up on your marketing before getting out there? This simple story illustrates the value of preparation. Some call it, work smart versus working hard.

It makes more sense to do your research and fashion strategies before racing off to promote your services. Your menu and pricing constitute strategic business-building tools. It's all about getting repeat business and attracting new customers.

Another classic mistake is underestimating the time it takes to build a customer base. I've witnessed this problem time and again. Business is slower than anticipated. I know, I'll drop my prices! That should drum up more appointments!

Flat rate, price drop - every day, business flop. Here's how the problem becomes intractable. That strategy only appeals to customers trawling for discounts and special offers. If you run flat rate specials every week, before you know it, you've dug yourself into a discount hole. The clients who respond to that sort of marketing will expect nothing less.

When you understand that your services attract a variety of customers, you can target them in different ways. Consequently, your business will function efficiently at different price ranges, all while promoting the massage services that most appeal to you.

DESIGNING YOUR MENU -
DIFFERENT TYPES OF CONSUMERS

First things first, draw up a list of the categories of services you can offer. Mind you, this is the research phase, nothing's set in stone.

This is just the creative process. Put your brain into overdrive and see if you can come up with some more ideas that would fit your business.

New customers, Spa package customers, Wellness Program customers, Membership customers, Coupon customers, Urgent scheduling,

Best deal customers, Celebration customers,

Specialty services, and Luxury packages

You want to identify these customers because you should market them differently. Resist the instinct to lump all advertising in one category.

For example, the price of a 60-minute massage is $75.00. New customer, same price.

Monthly customers, same price.

Slow season, same price.

If your busiest day of the week is Saturday, don't offer promotions on

Saturdays. Saturday should be the day you bring in the most money. Keep your discounts for your slow days.

Offering a variety of services allows you to target clients at different price points. It is smart marketing. Jump on this insight to build a successful, sustainable business.

DESIGN YOUR MENU - SPA PACKAGES

WHY OFFER SPA PACKAGES?

Depending on the services you include, you can earn more money within the same time period. Spa packages allow you to charge more for extra services and products.

Hot stone massage is an in-demand moneymaker. It's all about adding value to the same service.

There will be an initial investment to buy products for these value-added services. On the upside, they can be used repeatedly, with no further out-of-pocket expenses. The 60-minute session doesn't take any longer, you're just charging more for the allotted time on account of the enhanced service.

You can also allocate money to create luxury packages. Keep in mind, decadent, organic massage oils, body scrubs, polishes, and butter creams will be a bigger investment per session because those inputs aren't reusable. However, you can still make more money on the spa packages as the cost of those inputs will always be less than the price of the service. The use of such products gives you the flexibility to infuse your menu with more luxury offerings.

Always be mindful of the wording used to create your packages. Look at the difference between these three services.

- 60 minute massage $75.00
- 60 minute massage with hot stones $95.00
- Relaxation Package

Enjoy a 60-minute customized massage. Your massage package includes deep relaxing hot stones and a hot towel peppermint foot treatment. Melt your stress away with this massage package. Regular price $99.00 On Sale $79.00

If you were a potential customer mulling over these three options, which one would appeal to you? The package that offers more value attracts customers. The package that allows the customer to imagine the experience will attract more business.

Put your spa packages at higher prices. The higher price reflects the additional value and products included in the package. Customers want to feel they are getting good value for their dollars.

Higher prices also allow the business to adjust the sale price as business picks up. As your appointment book fills up, your sale prices change. Sale prices can increase without having to change your original menu price.

If your services start out at a higher price point, it allows your business to make more money without updating printed material or telling customers your prices are going up.

You can also promote the services that most tickle your fancy. If

Lavender Infusion Massage is your thing, then list that spa package on sale and keep the other spa packages at regular price.

Another benefit of higher priced spa package is gratuity. Many clients do a flat rate percentage. Higher prices will yield higher tips.

For more information on how to create spa packages please read my book:

Massage Marketing - Don't Leave Money On The Table Earn more money with an infusion of creative services to reel in more clients. www.MassageMarketing101.com

DESIGN YOUR MENU - FIRST TIME CUSTOMERS

Promotions are an effective way to reel in first timers. You can offer a special without applying a discount to every customer.

This new customer incentive can be fluid. You have the freedom to change the offer monthly. If there are several openings available, sweeten the new customer offer. If you are almost fully booked, fix the offer at a smaller discount. If you are able to access your website editing and online scheduling, it's easy to update the promotion of your new customer offer.

One great way to add value to a first-time client is with the inclusion of some of the tools or products that cost you little or nothing.

For example, if you've purchased hot stones, throw those in on the deal. This will amp up the value without an additional cost to you. If you have extra products you want to use, include those as well.

You may have a half-gallon of mango butter or peppermint sugar scrub products and they are approaching their expiration date. Create a package with a mango butter hydrating hand & foot treatment or peppermint sugar scrub treatment. That's an irresistible lure.

Set up a page on your website directed at new customers. Give potential new clients some insight into what they can expect when they visit your practice. If you're not keen on hard membership sales, include that information. Highlight your specialties. If you don't deduct 10 minutes for changing, share that.

Share information about your business with new customers so they get a feel for you. Remember, connecting with your customer is what creates relationships.

This new customer website page is the ideal place to include reviews highlighting unique features of your business or therapists. Start grooming client relationships with your customized website page.

Here's an easy way to format what your business offers.

Have a list of what new clients can expect or a Q & A section to address some of the common questions you get from potential new clients.

What to expect at (your business name here)?

Expect to work with an experienced massage therapist. Our therapists average 8 years in the field. Massage is a gamble; you never know what you'll get. You have a greater chance of having all your expectations met with a therapist who has more experience under their belt. Please arrive 10 minutes early for your first session in order to complete our client information form.

Expect your therapist to be attentive to your needs and to be quiet during your session. This is your time to relax and loosen tight and stressed muscles. We do not engage in talking.

Expect no upselling during or after your session.

Expect no sales pitch or membership selling.

At the end of your massage, you will receive a bottle of water and our profound gratitude for your business.

What people are saying about (your business name here)?

My massage therapist was so fantastic! I was gifted a massage gift card from my husband. I made an appointment when I had a stressful week at work.

I had quite a few knots in my back muscles but felt completely relaxed when all was done! I got the stone massage which was incredible. I will be back again. - Bethany

If you have online scheduling, create a tab or category for new customers.

Okay, so you're probably wondering, if someone books a 60-minute massage under the regular pricing, do you bring up your new customer discount?

Do you have to offer new customer specials to everyone new?

It's your call. Many businesses won't suggest discounts if the customer hasn't asked about them. They will charge the price of the service the customer booked.

One way to determine whether a customer is researching first timer offers is to have your new customer promotions a little different.

Have the name of the package unique or the length of service different.

Creating two new customer offers can be smart advertising.

For example, perhaps you offer a new customer an 80- minute massage. If your regular prices don't include 80 minutes, you'll know the person calling wants the new customer discount.

CREATE A SPA PACKAGE.

For example: Celebration Package - Enjoy a 50-minute massage with warm, relaxing hot stones. New Customer offer only $65.00. (Regular price $85.00)

By changing the length of service or creating a spa package for new customers, you'll know the customer who booked wants a discount. If a customer isn't searching for new customer discounts, they will book a basic 60 or 90-minute massage and pay regular prices.

DESIGN YOUR MENU - WELLNESS PROGRAMS OR

Let's examine another dimension of the massage therapy business; wellness programs.

WHY OFFER WELLNESS PROGRAMS? WHAT INSPIRES CUSTOMERS TO SIGN UP FOR SUCH PROGRAMS?

A price conscious consumer will examine your prices. If you offer a flat rate price for all your massages, there is no motivation to become a wellness customer.

WHY DO BUSINESSES WANT WELLNESS CUSTOMERS ANYWAY?

Wellness customers create loyalty. They are the definition of repeat business because wellness is a long-haul lifestyle choice. Developing relationships with clients can help businesses build and sustain long term success.

Repeat customers are beneficial for your business in many ways. They provide a dependable, consistent income stream. If your business has

50 customers on the wellness plan, that's 50 customers locked in each month.

One of the concerns with the massage industry or any service industry is low seasons or dry spells.

Research shows consumers spend more on massage therapy during certain months of the year. You have bills to pay regardless of the shifting sands of business fortunes. Repeat customers can give you much needed peace of mind with income you can count on.

Regular repeat customers also derive better health benefits under your hands. You become aware of their likes and dislikes, which enables you to tailor packages specifically for them. This leads to greater client satisfaction which will, in turn, strengthen your relationships.

A wellness program generates repeat business without hard sales pitches. The more value you create in your wellness plan, the more it motivates customers to get on board...or on the table.

You can offer different types of wellness plans. One way to go is a non-contract plan. This is an appealing option for a client nervous about being wedded to an agreement. Customers loathe manipulation and may have heard horror stories of customers who were sold into a 12-month deal with a massage business.

Clients often complain about some massage membership chain businesses. They feel as though they're perceived solely as a dollar sign and not a person. Here's the rub, a massage naturally releases feel-good hormones. After a massage, customers are riding the high of those happy hormones. Being pressed into a 12-month contract while under the influence of those feel-good hormones can leave the client with buyer's remorse.

Not all chain stores manipulate clients in this vulnerable state. The ones who do, however, create a negative impression of the industry among clients who come to feel like they've been played.

It's all down to communication. Customers can be turned off if a business is overly aggressive in trying to sell memberships. With a few wellness options in your arsenal, the customer can choose from your varied menu.

Some call this the soft sale. I call it "massaging the sale." Sorry, I couldn't help it!

You want to create a pressure-free environment, one that doesn't force an immediate decision.

It's a good idea to showcase the price benefits of wellness programs in your marketing materials. A framed flyer on your desk puts those benefits front and center where your customers can see them.

Here's another wonderful marketing tool to pollinate your customers' minds with wellness plans. Create business cards with your wellness plan printed on them. This is a terrific soft sale tool. Give each customer this business card. If it feels appropriate, take a few minutes to explain the options as you hand them the business card. This soft form of selling is sharing information without pressure to decide.

This is especially smart marketing if you have a therapist on staff who is a little timid. They can distribute the business cards without feeling pressured to close a membership sale.

If you would like me to send you a sample flyer, please email me at SabrinaTonneson@gmail.com. In the subject, request FREE flyer to promote wellness programs.

You can run promotions to get a big influx of wellness customers. For example, sign up for a six-month term and get a free 30-minute upgrade on the sixth month. Or, sign up for a six-month term and receive a free massage on the sixth month.

The more value you offer during the promotion, the greater the possibility of selling more memberships. If you want this promotion to be a one-time affair - use the words "Introductory Offer". This lets your customers know if they re-enroll in another six-month term, they won't be receiving the promotional offer again.

DESIGN YOUR MENU - HOW TO CREATE A MEMBERSHIP CONTRACT

There are no hard rules for contracts. You can customize them as you see fit.

Some businesses don't offer wellness plans because they're reluctant to wrangle with contracts and cancellations. The advent of the "bad online review" has made massage therapy businesses leery of contract arrangements. The last thing they want is a disgruntled customer burning the midnight oil on the internet to burn their business reputation.

It needn't be that way.

If a customer wants to cancel, you can decide how to handle it individually. If there's no interest in keeping them shackled to the contract, simply tell that customer you'll allow a one-time, penalty-free cancellation.

The reason a contract is beneficial, even if you don't plan to enforce it, is because it convinces your customers to come in monthly. You create a mutually beneficial exchange. They get the best prices, you get regular monthly customers.

If you have a wellness customer unable to keep their appointments, you can customize the arrangement. You can decide how you want to proceed case by case.

Worst-case scenario, you've processed two months of payments, but they never came in. Now, they are calling to say they want out and a refund.

Refunds are a headache for most businesses as they incur fees and extra paperwork.

One easy solution can be to tell your customer you will allow them to can cancel without penalties. Explain that you won't bill them for the balance of their contract. Let them know they will have an in-store credit of _ dollars.

If they're unable to come in, they can gift their store credit to a friend. The friend can use the store credit toward regular price services.

You always want to appear accommodating and non-confrontational. Instead of saying, "no, you signed a contract that says no refunds", outline what you can do for them. This is a customer service 101 tip.

Remember, if you have a customer asking for something and you are not sure how to respond immediately, tell them you need to discuss it with your partner. (Some people think if they operate the business alone they have no partner. A partner can be someone who is your sounding board. They can be a silent partner. They can be an emotional, supportive partner. You do not have to disclose who is your partner or partners.) You can tell them you will call them back in a day. Take some time and think about how you want to handle the situation.

If you would like me to send you a copy of a sample contract, please email me at SabrinaTonneson@gmail.com. In the subject, write sample contract.

DESIGN YOUR MENU - MASSAGE THERAPY ENHANCEMENTS

It's a common theme in this book; variety is the spice of life. Additional menu options can enhance your profits.

You can create more menu options with add-ons or a la carte options. Some businesses call them massage therapy enhancements.

To help explain this concept, think of a restaurant menu. Most menus offer the option of purchasing items a la carte. This gives the customer the option to customize the massage with enhancements of their choice. One great way to advertise your enhancements is to list them on a flyer prominently displayed in the room where customers fill out paperwork.

To spotlight your massage therapy enhancements, you can offer a regular price service with one FREE enhancement of their choice. When a customer comes in, you can hand them a laminated list of enhancements to review and select one. This will clue them in on the extra services your business offers.

Sample ideas you can use to create your own laminated flyer.

MASSAGE THERAPY ENHANCEMENTS

Kansa Face Massage $15.00

Enjoy a slow relaxing face massage, which uses Kansa handheld contouring tool to balance the Ayurvedic doshas. Tightens and tones skin.

Face Mask $15.00

Deep cleaning clay face mask, followed by aromatherapy warm face towels. Includes moisturizing face massage. Great to clear sinuses, and opens energy channels in the face.

Deep Tissue Cupping on Back $15.00

Massage cupping works deeper by loosening adhesions, facilitating the muscles to operate more independent.

Cupping stimulates the skin by increasing circulation while separating fused tissue layer and draining lymph. Massage cupping can leave "hickey"-like marks on skin.

Hot Stone Foot Treatment $15.00

Warm relaxing hot towels foot wrap followed by hot stone foot massage. Soothes, hydrates and refreshes tired feet.

Hot Oil Scalp Massage $15.00

Hot moisturizing oils of jojoba, grapeseed, sesame, apricot and aloe vera used to massage scalp. Hot oil scalp massage feels fabulous and can help with dry skin or hair loss.

Muscle & Joint Therapy $15.00

Therapeutic massage for aching muscles and sore joints. Massage creme includes natural botanicals to help reduce inflammation, followed by cooling pain relief polar lotion. Polar lotion relaxes muscles with oils of wintergreen, peppermint and aloe.

Hot Stones $15.00

Warm relaxing hot stones help to release tension from tight and sore muscles. Heated hot stones help you to go into a deep state of relaxation.

Pick one targeted muscle group 1) neck/back 2) legs/feet or 3) arms/hands

WHAT ARE SOME ADDITIONAL MASSAGE THERAPY ENHANCEMENTS OPTIONS?

- Massage Face Cupping
- Asian Spoon Face Massage
- Gua Sha Massage
- Kansa Wand Contouring Sugar Scrub
- Peppermint Masque Foot Treatment
- Hands & Feet Shea Butter Moisturizing Treatment
- Cold Stone Therapy
- Salt Stones

Urgent Scheduling - extend your hours to accommodate client (some therapists will accommodate clients and come in after hours and charge after-hour rates)

To get more ideas - browse spa menu websites on the Internet.

DESIGN YOUR MENU - BIRTHDAY OFFERS

One great marketing tool is to offer birthday specials. If you know your customer's birthdate, you can email them birthday greetings and make them a birthday massage offer.

If you don't collect birthdate information, no worries. You can create a page on your website especially for birthday massage offers.

However, be on the lookout for the fake birthdays, clients trying to scam a promotional offer. To get around that, politely ask the client to show photo ID at the time of the appointment to verify the birth date.

There are many ways to create birthday offers. For your regular monthly customers, you might want to gift them with something even more extravagant, for example, a free 30-minute upgrade. This way you'll still earn some money on the appointment.

Some businesses will gift a whole session to their regulars. It depends on your business. Usually the customers who are gifted with either a free 30-minute upgrade or free 60-minute massage tip very high at that appointment. It helps breed loyalty when customers feel valued.

Another basic way to give regular or new customers a birthday gift is to offer a great package for them, perhaps a 75-minute massage with aromatherapy scalp massage, peppermint hot towel wrap and warm relaxing hot stones. Regular price $129.00 - Birthday special $69.00!

You can stipulate a specific time within which the birthday customer must use this offer. This could be 15 days before or after their birth date. That gives the customer a 30-day window to get their appointment scheduled.

Couples massage is another great idea for birthdays as someone is usually treating the birthday person. The birthday couples massage allows them to enjoy the gift together. It's a fun activity to share and they get to shed some stress in the bargain.

DESIGN YOUR MENU - REFERRALS

DO YOU OFFER REFERRALS? WHAT ARE THE
BENEFITS? HOW CAN YOU USE REFERRALS TO BUILD
YOUR BUSINESS QUICKLY?

First of all, referrals are one of the best marketing tools bar none! The reason referrals are marketing gold is because the new customer already feels they will be satisfied. Remember, massage is a gamble. When you go to a new business, you can't predict the experience. You can't be sure if you'll like the location, the atmosphere, the staff or the style of massage.

If someone has recommended a therapist or a business, that recommendation removes risk as it is an endorsement by someone who has already sampled the goods. So how can you reward customers who do the advertising for you?

First, recognize that advertising costs money. It's better to invest your money on guaranteed customers rather than maybe customers. There's no reward for a referral unless a customer comes in, whereas with advertising, you pay for ads regardless of how much business comes your way.

The other benefit of referrals is you show your customers you value and appreciate their word of mouth recommendations.

One great way to get your customers to invest time and energy promoting your business is to offer a new customer special, and then give the client making the referrals a reward.

Some will offer a $10.00 in-store credit for each referral.

One business owner I mentored decided to offer a whole session, a 60-minute massage for each referral. Her regular prices are higher than average price. For example, she charges $95.00 for 60 minutes instead of the $75.00 going rate in her area. Even though her prices were higher than average, she created extra value for her customers.

She takes her time with each customer and often gives

him or her an extra 5 to 10 minutes. She does a wonderful intake/communication before each session starts, therefore, she is able to customize and deliver what the client is looking for. She includes the extras in her treatment, without any up charges. She has raving customers who are more than excited to tell their friends and family. Her business grew quickly with her one free massage for each referral program. She consistently does 10 appointments per week (her goal), and she's booked out several weeks in advance. She has the 'reward creates reward' down to a science!

One idea to accelerate business growth is to offer a temporary referral promotion. Let's say your normal reward for referrals is one free therapy enhancement. You can offer: for the month of (whatever the month is) all referrals receive 1 Free Therapy Enhancement and $20.00 in-store credit. If a customer refers 3 friends who come in that month - they will have an instore credit of $60.00 and 3 Free Therapy Enhancements to use.

This can encourage customers to talk to their friends, family and co-workers. It creates momentum!

The bigger the promotions or offer you make, the greater the incentive for your clients to get out there and sing your praises. You can have a contest. Offer a discount for each referral, and a free massage for the client who brings in the most referrals during the specified time.

This, again, can encourage customers to go and sell your business. Some people enjoy the challenge of winning and will be motivated to go get you those referral customers.

DESIGN YOUR MENU - LOYALTY REWARD PROGRAM

Loyalty is a highly valued commodity in the massage therapy business. It's a trait you'll definitely want to honor in your customers. There are several ways you can do that.

If you create loyalty reward business cards, they might put the card in their wallets. They will see the card randomly and recall how much they enjoy your massages. The business card is a visual reminder.

Loyalty rewards show your customers you acknowledge their importance to your business. It's also a great selling tool. Some people may forget you offer a loyalty program, particularly if it isn't printed on your menu or highlighted on your website.

If a client received their 3rd massage, you tell them with their next massage that they get their reward (provided you offer rewards on every 4th massage).

This motivates people to schedule sooner rather than later as everyone loves a reward!

HERE ARE SOME SAMPLE IDEAS OF LOYALTY REWARDS.

- Buy 3 massages get free 15-minute upgrade on 4th.
- Buy 3 massages get a free enhancement on 4th massage.
- Buy 3 massages get 4th massage half off.
- Buy 5 massages get 6th one free.
- Buy 5 massages and receive 30-minute free upgrade on your 6th massage.

(They would pay for 60 minutes but they would receive 90 minutes)

FINANCIAL GOALS

As you work on your marketing game, you always want to keep your financial targets in your sights. What are your basic needs, expenses and financial goals?

Business owners work backwards. That means you come up with your end total first, and then figure out how to create the sum.

For example, if your basic income need is $500.00 a week, $500.00 is going to be the sum. Next you create formulas and strategies to get to that figure.

Most businesses have 2 or 3 sum goals. The first sum total covers the bare minimum, that's just the scratch to pay your overhead.

The next dollar goal will be higher, your average sum. It includes the bare basics and some extra dollars to give you a bit of wiggle room. Wiggle room includes money for unexpected expenses as well as rainy-day savings for slow periods.

Your 3rd sum total will be your financial success goal. This total will reflect revenues to think big with business upgrades, a bonus for yourself, or that miniature donkey you've had your eye on for some time; whatever your mind can conjure. (smile)

These sum totals and goals will change over time.

Smart businesses re-evaluate their sum totals and goals every 90 days.

How much do you need to earn a week to meet your sum goals?

Bare basic sum goal? _____

Average sum goal? _____

Financial success goal? _____

EVALUATING THE CURRENT STATE OF YOUR BUSINESS

Continually take the pulse of your massage therapy operation.

How is your business currently operating?

If you already have clients, let's examine what percentage of your business is already filled.

How many appointments a week can your business offer?

How many appointments a week is your business averaging?

If your business can do 50 appointments a week, and you're averaging 10 appointments a week, you have an 80% opportunity for growth.

What percentage of growth is available for your business?

Now we want to cross-reference our sum totals with your existing income.

How much income are you currently averaging per week?

If your 10 appointments are averaging $700.00 a week and your basic sum is $500.00/week, your business is in a great place for growth without stress.

A calculation of the numbers will help determine the health and prospects for your business. It's important to know the current state of your business.

An assessment will help you determine how much vigor you apply to marketing and promotions. If your business is in crisis mode, there will be more of an incentive to offer bigger promotions. You will also want to invest more time in marketing. If you are currently investing 2 hours a week marketing - passing out flyers, posting on social media, etc. You might want to invest 3 or 4-hours marketing. Temporally invest more time in marketing.

One problem that some businesses experience is they've not planned their marketing and financial strategy. The business is not earning enough to pay the overhead and panic ensues.

The typical panic response is price cuts for all services. It's possible to oversaturate customers with regular discounted specials. This can hurt the business because now the customers expect to only pay the discounted prices.

Understanding the power of pricing is crucial. Learning how to strategically offer discounts and designing thoughtful menus is important to the health of your business.

If your business is currently struggling, it's not too late. You can restructure your operation and attract new customers as well as create different relationships with existing customers who only pay discounted prices.

For example, you can turn your price conscious customer into a wellness plan customer.

RESEARCH AND RAISING PRICES

Next, let's gather some information. If you haven't already researched other businesses, now is the time.

Google 'massage' and scrutinize massage businesses in your area. Call each business or scout their websites. Research chiropractors, fitness centers and day spas as well. Make notes of each business and their prices. You also want to study their menus. Do they offer a variety of services? Do they have a specialty service? Do they have a signature massage package? Do they have wellness or membership programs? You want to ingest and analyze all of this information.

One business owner felt uncomfortable raising her prices until she did this homework. She was shocked to discover other businesses charged over $20.00 more for the same services. She realized if she raised her prices, she could save for a much-needed vacation. She also got excited about upgrades she could buy for her business.

Prices can have a psychological effect on owners. Many make the mistake of assuming the price of the service is what they earn per hour. They forget to factor in all the hours that go into operating the business. Hours invested in marketing, researching, accounting, cleaning, managing, social media connections, customer service, appointment setting, etc.

If you track all the hours you invest in your business each week, including the time you deliver the hands-on massage, you'll work out what you really earn per hour.

Most business owners often get an unpleasant surprise when they take the time to calculate their real hourly wage.

One business owner I consulted with was apprehensive about raising her prices. We develop a strategy to allow her regular customers to be grandfathered in for 6 months at existing prices, while new customers paid the new prices. She had never considered the idea she could raise prices for new customers and allow specific clients to keep current prices.

Yes. Business owners can customize their pricing. Create strategies that make it easy for you to raise your prices.

SAMPLE MENU PLAN

I've got some homework for you.

What is the average price in your area? _____

What is your lowest price you're willing to accept for a customer who signs a contract or buys a package of 6 or more? _____

Are you willing to add services to your menu? _____

Will you be using therapy enhancements to create packages or offer add-ons? _____

Are you going to offer a promotional reward (temporary or permanent) for referrals? _____

How fast do you want to grow your business? _____

The faster you want to grow your business, the more promotions you'll want to offer. This is a great time to make temporary offers.

Example: one-month big rewards for referrals. ($25.00 store credit for each referral)

One-month promotion, offer great prices on package of 3 (to be used in

3 months or some expiration that is sooner rather than later - perhaps allow the package to be shared with friends/family).

Do you plan to have more appointment slots available in the near future? (Perhaps hiring more staff or adding more hours yourself)

This is a sample homework.

20 slots available a week - currently filling 10 slots each week. Average price in my area $65.00/hour

Therapist is currently charging $60.00/hour.

The lowest price therapist is willing to work is $55.00/hour

Yes, to adding a variety of items on menu.

Yes, to temporary offers to grow business faster.

This is a sample pricing and menu for the above sample homework results.

Raise price from $60.00 per hour to $69.00 per hour.

Contact regular customers and let them know you are raising your prices. You can grandfather them in at same prices for 3 months or longer. Customers can be offered the option to be on a monthly wellness plan without prepaying or signing a contract. You can customize any arrangement that works for you. Make sure you are clear on the details.

One business owner I mentored had a few monthly clients. She told them she would grandfather them in with the original price. She never told them they would need to keep coming in monthly to keep the agreement active, nor did she give them a timeline for the agreement.

Fast forward, some of those customers stopped coming in regularly. When they do come in, they wanted the original price. This business owner is now very busy with higher paying customers, but she honors the price with those customers. She learned an important lesson: get clear on the details, before you make an offer to someone.

SAMPLE MENU

Regular Price

$69.00 per hour

New Customer Special

60-minute massage plus one massage therapy enhancement of their choice.

Only $59.00

Regular price for this service is $69.00 for massage and $15.00 for the complimentary enhancement upgrade = $84.00 (New customers save $25.00)

Wellness Programs

Option 1 - Return within 30 days and automatically get $5.00 off. No contract.

Option 2 - 3-month term $60.00 each (prepay $180.00 or charge their credit card on the 1st of each month)

Option 3 - 12-month term $55.00 each - (prepay or charge their credit card monthly)

Spa Packages: Pick names and content for each spa package.

Relaxation Package

60-minute massage with deep relaxing hot stones, aromatherapy scalp massage and hot towels - regular price $99.00

On Sale $75.00

Tranquility Package

75-minute customized massage, including warm relaxing hot stones, hot oil scalp massage and deep moisturizing peppermint, shea butter hand and foot massage - regular price $149.00

On Sale $99.00

Ten Dollar Tuesdays

All services are $10.00 off on Tuesdays.

(Not Valid for Wellness Customers)

Referral Program

$10.00 in store credit for each person a client refers.

This menu and new prices actually allow the business owner to earn more money. She's only offering her lowest prices to the customers who will come in monthly with a twelve-month agreement. She no longer offers a flat rate $60.00 massage.

This new price structure generates more business and more profits as she is able to target to a larger audience.

She'll take a temporary loss on the in-store referral credit, but she will be getting new customers without coming out of pocket to advertise. She will also be deducting the in-store credit from her new higher price of $69.00 instead of $60.00. She will be creating relationships and loyalty with her new and existing clients.

Tuesdays is her slow days and she averaged 1 appointment. She will take a slight loss on Tuesdays, but she is happy to have her one slow day booked. As her schedule becomes busier, she may change her Tuesday offer.

PRICING AND MENU WORKSHEET

Research at least 5 other businesses' prices and menus.

- Business
- Name
- 60 min price
- 90 min price
- Membership Program?
- New Customer Offer?
- Spa Packages?

Menu Options: Write your prices and create options. Delete or cross out what you don't want to include.

Add your own ideas. Once you get an overall sense of what services you want to offer and what prices you want to charge, create your own customized menu.

Massage Prices (pick how many options you want to offer).

- 30 minutes
- 45 minutes

- 50 minutes
- 60 minutes
- 75 minutes
- 80 minutes
- 90 minutes

Specialty Services (can include sports massage, couples massage, reiki energy, work, lymphatic treatments, pregnancy etc.).

New Customer Offer

(Pick if you want 1 or 2 new customer offers. Good idea is to have a shorter service for lower price and longer service for higher price. This will allow two different types of customers to book.)

- Option 1
- Option 2

WELLNESS PLANS (MEMBERSHIP)

Option 1 - return in 30 days no contract

- 50 or 60-minute price?
- 80 or 90-minute price?

Option 2 - six-month term (paid at beginning of each month or prepaid package - create what you want to offer)

- 50 or 60-minute price?
- 80 or 90-minute price?

Customize your own wellness offer

Spa Packages (create different lengths of time with different enhancements upgrades included)

- Option 1
- Option 2
- Option 3

Massage Therapy Enhancements – Add–ons

Referral Program

Loyalty Program

SUCCESS STORIES

When Sabrina suggested I add a menu to my business, I didn't think it would be useful. I rent a room in a professional building and I work for myself. I decided to try it and, to my surprise, I noticed a difference right away.

My new customer offer was a hit and I received a big influx of new customers. My birthday offer is another big hit. I found more and more of my clients recommending me to their friends.

I make more money now.

My most popular service is the 60-minute Lavender Infusion package where my customers get hot stones and aromatherapy. Customers love this package and I make more money for this session!

Plus, I have almost 20 people who are on my wellness plan. I am staying busy, even during slow times.

I really underestimated how much value I would receive by offering a menu. I am so happy I tried it! Menus are one of the best-kept secrets in the therapeutic massage industry. - Carol Jons LMT

I work for myself out of my home. When Sabrina encouraged me to bring in a menu for my services, I felt silly. Menus are for bigger businesses and day spas.

I was skeptical, so I decided to start with only 3 items on the menu. 1. New Customer offer 2. Ultimate Relaxation offer (90-minute massage with all the extras) and 3. Package of 3 (prepaid package).

I typed up my menu and I started to hand it out to customers, as well as I started to leave my menu around town. The first few weeks I didn't notice a change, but then I started getting calls about the new customer offer. Some of my regulars decided to upgrade and try the Ultimate Relaxation package. I would say over 50% of them continue to book that package now.

I am seeing results with this menu. I am going to expand my menu again and give my existing customers and potential new customers more options. I really like this marketing plan. - Jan Blanshan - LMT

We already had a list of services when I hired Sabrina for consulting. Working with Sabrina, we realized we were not making the extra money for upgrades because our staff was already including upgrades for free in the basic massage service.

We needed to restructure to get everyone on same page. I hired Sabrina to lead a meeting with my staff. She was able to professionally articulate the importance of everyone being on same page. She motivated the therapists to want to sell upgrades and gave demonstrations on how to get upgrades without sounding pushy.

One example is to offer a customer a one-time sample of an upgrade. We gave the therapists bonuses for selling upgrades. This extra income encouraged the therapists to sell the upgrades.

After the staff meeting, I noticed a difference. First, our staff is now aware it is not okay to offer the extras if the customer is not paying.

We are seeing more and more upgrades. Sabrina suggested we offer a game for upgrade sales. Not a competition game between the therapists, but a game where everyone can be a winner. If therapist sold 5 or more upgrades a week - they got a bonus $10.00 gift card to Starbucks. The therapists all love their coffee! If they sold 9 or more upgrades a week, they got a $20.00 gift card. We played this game for 3 consecutive weeks and we noticed each week therapists were selling more and more. Everyone was a winner.

It was a genius idea as it really helped the therapists get comfortable talking about upgrades. Now, our regular customers are requesting upgrades on their own as they love them!

I highly recommend calling in support. It is wonderful to have an outside person come in with new eyes and offer insights as well as motivation. Thanks

Sabrina! You clearly love massage and business; your passion is contagious! - Vicky Dale - LMT

CONSULTATIONS

Sabrina is available for consultations. Consultations are a wonderful tool for any individual business or company.

Hire Sabrina today and get help with any of the following.

- Increase profits
- Feeling stuck
- Staff problems or challenges
- Take your business to next level
- Get more customers
- Need motivation
- Customizing your menu and prices
- Create new marketing strategies
- Hiring
- Customer service
- Staff training
- Growing pains
- Team energy and harmonizing

For more information and a special offer, please go to www.MassageMarketing101.com

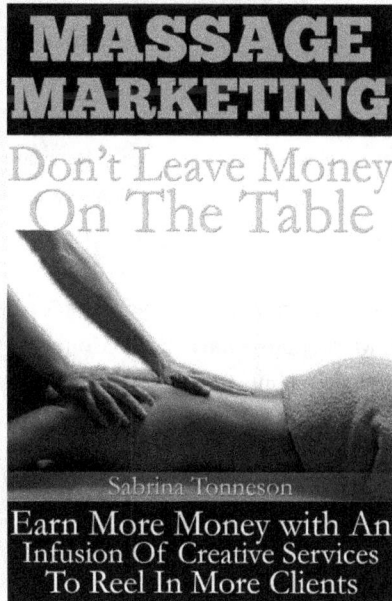

MASSAGE MARKETING – DON'T LEAVE MONEY ON THE TABLE

You've got the expertise and your customer service is on point. All that's missing is that imaginative spark to set you apart from other massage therapists. Massage Marketing – Don't Leave Money on the Table is that missing link to help you create unique spa packages that snag the attention of more clients.

- Earn 30% more with the addition of creative spa packages
- Dynamic ideas to create attractive services that will lure additional clientele
- Catchy names to make your massage offerings stand out

- Tips and tools to structure your profit-spinning product menu

Once you've settled on a menu to ensure you're charging the right price for your invaluable services, the next step is to fill that menu with creative packages that will captivate your clients and grow your business.

Hawaiian Escape, Lavender Infusion, this book is filled with ideas for seductive packages that tell clients what you bring to the massage table goes well beyond a deep tissue massage. With Massage Marketing - Don't Leave Money on the Table, you'll learn all the strategies to create an unforgettable massage experience that offers a world of options to clients looking for something exotic and adventurous. Go from back-rub to Bali bliss, and spark the imagination of your clients. With the help of this book, soon they will want to try every journey into nirvanic bliss you've added to your diverse menu. Order Massage Marketing - Don't Leave Money on the Table now and transform your practice into a temple of alluring tranquility and business prosperity.

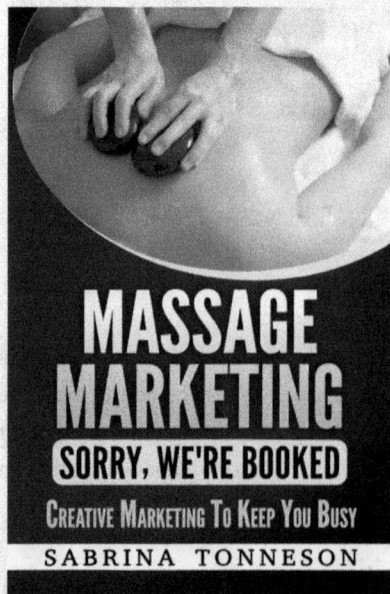

MASSAGE MARKETING
SORRY, WE'RE BOOKED
CREATIVE MARKETING TO KEEP YOU BUSY
SABRINA TONNESON

SORRY – WE'RE BOOKED

- Book covers low cost or free marketing strategies
- Pick up techniques to attract a broader customer base
- Learn the art of the subtle sale that wins new clients
- Convince existing customers to maintain regular bookings

Sorry, we're booked." Those words are like a warm hug for any business owner. It suggests your livelihood is on the up. That's precisely the intent of this marketing book, to create that euphoric state of being busy in business. With the principles and guidelines contained in my course, you'll learn strategies you can immediately employ to bump up sales and bring more clients through the door. Whether you're a bespoke suit maker or a travel consultant, Sorry, We're Booked is chock-full of broadly applicable techniques that can turbo charge the revenues of any business. Worried that your limited marketing budget isn't up to the challenge of meeting your business goals? This structured marketing class explores effective techniques that are either low cost or free, costing you nothing but time and a bit of creative thinking!

My easy-to-follow course focuses on the subtleties of seduction marketing; you'll discover how to sweep customers off their feet with a soft-touch sales pitch. Sign up for this course now and savor the feeling of uttering those words, "Sorry, we're booked."

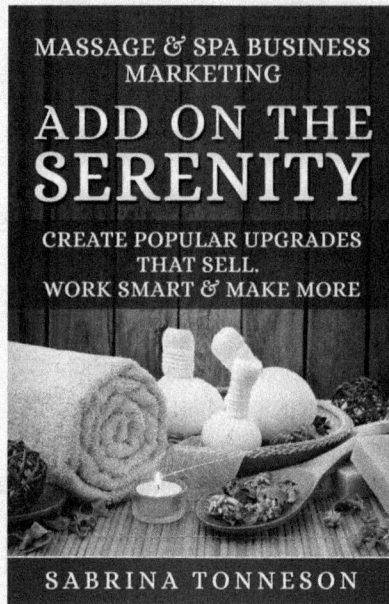

MASSAGE & SPA BUSINESS MARKETING

ADD ON THE SERENITY

CREATE POPULAR UPGRADES THAT SELL.
WORK SMART & MAKE MORE

SABRINA TONNESON

MASSAGE MARKETING - ADD ON THE SERENITY

A smart way to earn more money from massage therapy and spa services. Are you a professional that specializes in massage therapy, spa services, bodywork or energy healing? Why miss the opportunity to earn more and work less, while offering new exciting experiences to your clients?

Add on The Serenity book is a practical guide to creating an upgrade menu and selling upgrades.

- Upgrade options
- Upgrades for dry treatment rooms
- Body upgrades *Face upgrades
- Outside the box upgrades
- Create powerful descriptions
- Pricing
- Upgrades that sell

- Promoting Upgrades

When given the choice between getting less and getting more, people will always choose more. That's what an upgrade is: for your client, it's a chance to get additional services they probably never realized they wanted, needed, or could get. For you, it's the chance to earn more. It's what we call a win-win! In this book, you will learn how to capitalize on the idea of "more", offer service upgrades and add-ons, run promotions, and, of course, earn more without having to work more! So, What Are You Still Waiting For?

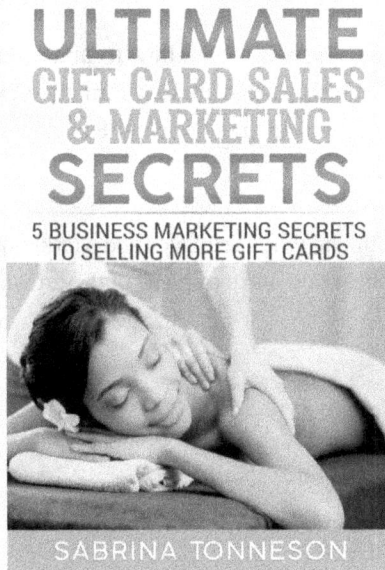

ULTIMATE
GIFT CARD SALES
& MARKETING
SECRETS
5 BUSINESS MARKETING SECRETS
TO SELLING MORE GIFT CARDS

SABRINA TONNESON

THE ULTIMATE GIFT CARD SALES & MARKETING SECRETS

Turbo Charge Your Gift Card Sales and Marketing with 5 Revenue-Boosting Secrets.

Up your game and boost revenues in the gift cards sales arena with the invaluable wisdom contained in this one-of-a-kind book. Don't leave your business marketing success to fate.

In 2015, gift card sales in the United States amounted to an estimated 130 billion U.S. dollars. The trends point to further upward growth in the popularity of this consumer electronic pass to convenience and value. This gift card sales and marketing book helps you take advantage of the surging trends with some inside knowledge that puts you ahead of the game. With some easy-to-apply-steps you can learn how to avoid underpricing, achieve year-round sales, create gift card terms for profit and create campaigns to stimulate buyer interest and rack up those sales.

This book is structured with an easy-to-follow format and is bursting at the margins with tips and techniques that are transformative for both the aspiring sales and marketing entrepreneur and the seasoned business marketing dealmaker.

Order your copy of Ultimate Gift Card Sales and Marketing Secrets and learn the strategies that can help you make a splash in the growing gift card sales market.

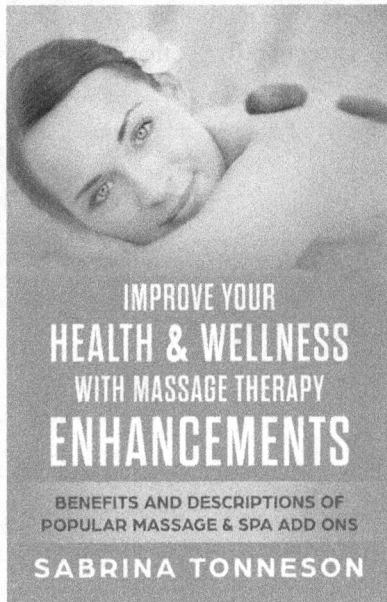

IMPROVE YOUR HEALTH & WELLNESS WITH MASSAGE THERAPY ENHANCEMENTS: BENEFITS AND DESCRIPTIONS OF POPULAR MASSAGE & SPA ADD ON THERAPIES

- Boost your massage therapy business revenues with diverse options for alluring massage packages
- Learn the descriptions and benefits of different massage therapies to try at home

Perhaps you'd like to explore the full potential of your massage therapy business. This book offers you an innovative range of options for alluring massage and spa add-on therapies that will build loyalty among your clientele while, at the same time, growing it.

Maybe you'd like to discover new methods of massage therapies to try with loved ones at home. If there's one publication focused on holistic health through the undeniable power of different massage add ons, this is it.

Benefits and descriptions of 12 unique and progressive massage therapies:

- Basalt Hot Stone Massage
- Bamboo Therapy
- Jade Face Roller
- Himalayan Salt Stones
- Massage Cupping
- Kansa Wand
- Massage Blading
- Marble Cold Stone Massage
- Hot Stone Foot Massage
- Dry Brushing
- Sugar Scrub
- Thai Herbal Ball

This book honors the ancient traditions and medical benefits of massage therapy that dates back thousands of years. It looks to the treasured past while keeping an eye firmly on the future of new massage treatment techniques that deliver compelling results.

Improve Your Health & Wellness with Massage Therapy Enhancements not only teaches creative massage therapies, it outlines the specific health benefits to be derived from each tried and true method. This book will equip you with the knowledge and know-how to suggest therapies depending on the specific client needs.

Order your copy of Improve Your Health & Wellness with Massage Therapy Enhancements today and seize the power of invaluable health with your own hands.